Book
of
Sayings

PETA ZAFIR

Book of Sayings

Book 4

©2021 Peta Zafir

All rights reserved.

No part of this book may be reproduced in any form or by any electronic or mechanical means, including information storage and retrieval systems, without written permission from the author, except in the case of a reviewer, who may quote brief passages embodied in critical articles or in a review.

Trademarked names appear throughout this book. Rather than use a trademark symbol with every occurrence of a trademarked name, names are used in an editorial fashion, with no intention of infringement of the respective owner's trademark.

The information in this book is distributed on an "as is" basis, without warranty. Although every precaution has been taken in the preparation of this work, neither the author nor the publisher shall have any liability to any person or entity with respect to any loss or damage caused or alleged to be caused directly or indirectly by the information contained in this book.

Peta Zafir Publishing
www.petazafir.com

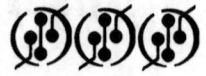

ISBN 978-0-6452140-6-2

Peta Zafir Publishing
www.petazafir.com
Peta Zafir You Tube Channel

BOOKS BY PETA ZAFIR

Health in Poetry Book 1
Health in Poetry Book 2
Book of Sayings Book 1
Book of Sayings Book 2
Book of Sayings Book 3
Book of Sayings Book 4
Scenar For Beginners

All books are available in print and eBook format from:
www.petazafir.com/books

Dedication

I dedicate this book to my third child and daughter Rebecca who taught me what feminism and personal choice is all about: honest, loving, caring, strong, focused and determined, plus the true personification of the Mother Earth woman.

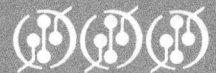

Book of Sayings   Book 4

Be the Woman that you Want Your

Daughter to Become

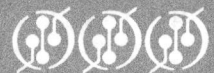

Book of Sayings   Book 4

Love is inherent

Racism, fear and hatred are taught

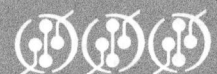

Book of Sayings   Book 4

Join Life Today
Be a part of something unbelievable
Get involved
Push your boundaries and
Face your own limitations

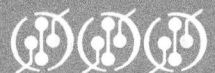

Book of Sayings   Book 4

We need to incorporate
All that Has Been
All that Exists Now, and
All that is Still Yet to Come

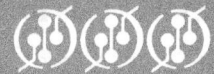

Book of Sayings   Book 4

Live Life, Study and Travel
Find your Place, Work Hard
Dare to Fail and Be brave
Make Decisions and Walk Forward and
Above all Keep Learning

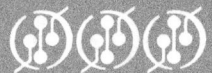

Book of Sayings   Book 4

Rejoice in the good times
Be proud of your achievements

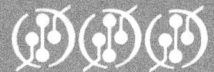

Book of Sayings   Book 4

You are unique and wonderful
Live that life
Be your own person
And Start NOW

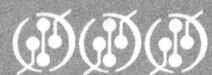

Book of Sayings   Book 4

Tell your Truth with compassion
gentleness and good faith

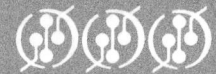

You are not responsible for another
person's happiness or sadness
And others are not responsibly for yours

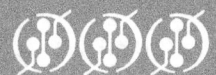

Book of Sayings   Book 4

Take responsibility for your life
Your emotional health and
Your physical wellbeing
You are your best advocate

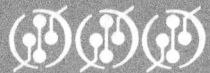

BOOK OF SAYINGS   BOOK 4

Stay true to yourself, and
Be open to learn and work hard

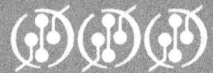

Book of Sayings   Book 4

Never give up on your Dreams

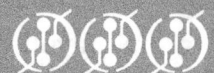

Book of Sayings   Book 4

To be true to yourself takes courage
It requires you to be introspective, sincere
open-minded and fair, and
Respectful and considerate of yourself

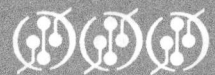

You are the leader of your life

Take charge

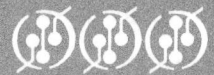

Book of Sayings   Book 4

You may choose not to be connected to
the family you are born into
You can create a family that you choose

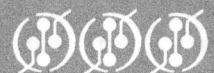

Book of Sayings   Book 4

Endings, Even when Welcomed
Have Sadness Connected to them

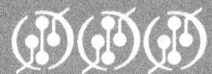

Book of Sayings   Book 4

Your Mind is a very powerful tool

Guard it well

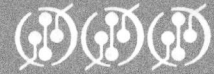

Book of Sayings   Book 4

Step forward
Life has a plan
We don't always know it
Yet it will unfold

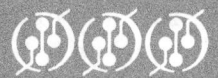

Book of Sayings   Book 4

When adversity comes
Fight on and don't question why
Work through it
Grow because of it
Learn as a result of it
This makes you the person
you were meant to be

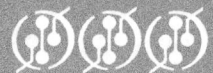

Book of Sayings   Book 4

The Past cannot be changed
Clear the issues
Release the baggage
Let them go and
Step forward

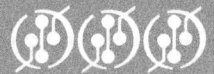

Book of Sayings   Book 4

If you worry and fret over
What will be
What will happen
What may occur
What if ...
Then you are living in the future
Allow life to unfold in its own time

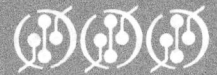

Book of Sayings   Book 4

Speak, act and live today
Live your life without Regrets

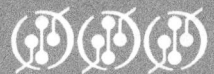

Learning who I was born to Be
through self-awareness, understanding
and acceptance
Empowers me to shine my Power

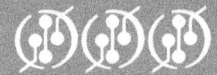

Book of Sayings   Book 4

If you want change
Change your behaviour
If you want a different life
Change your decisions and
If you want a different future
Change your present path

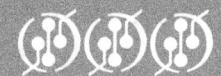

BOOK OF SAYINGS   BOOK 4

You are the guardian of your Power
Don't give it away, Guard it
Develop it and Step into it

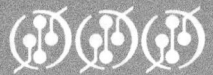

Book of Sayings   Book 4

Clear the Past and
Step into the Future

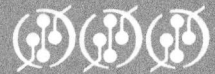

Book of Sayings   Book 4

Every day is a new beginning

Every experience is a new learning

Every choice is a new restarting

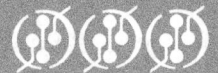

Book of Sayings   Book 4

Remember like any muscle
You need to work on Yourself
Over and over to become strong

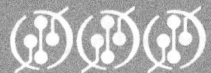

Book of Sayings   Book 4

Keep living well
Loving strong and
Being kind to yourself

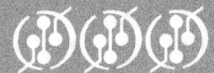

Book of Sayings   Book 4

There is always a Path
sometimes it just needs it illuminated

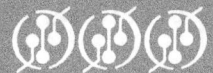

Book of Sayings   Book 4

Through hardships comes the light
Live in the light

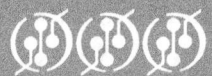

Happiness is not defined by the size of your house
your car, your wage, your job, your clothes
your partner, your suburb, your school, or your friends
Happiness is a choice within you

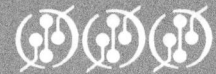

Book of Sayings   Book 4

When you are relaxed in yourself
Content with who you are
What you have and
Where you are going
You have Happiness present

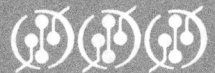

Book of Sayings   Book 4

Give where you can

without judgment or expectation

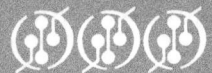

Happiness cannot be
Taken from you or given to you
It is yours to have freely and completely
Appreciate what you have and
Happiness will be the Gift you gain

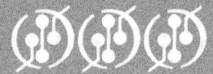

Book of Sayings   Book 4

There comes a time in one's life
Where we must understand our past
Take responsibility for our present and
Create the future we deserve

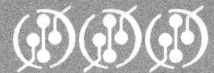

Book of Sayings   Book 4

Take hold of your future and never give the responsibility of your future to someone or something else

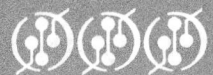

Book of Sayings   Book 4

Compassion and Connection

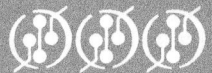

Book of Sayings   Book 4

Consistency is the winner
NOT Perfection

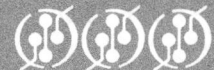

Book of Sayings   Book 4

Follow your path
Look for the opportunities and
Decide which are best for You

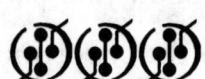

Peta Zafir Publishing
www.petazafir.com
Peta Zafir You Tube Channel

BOOKS BY PETA ZAFIR

Health in Poetry Book 1
Health in Poetry Book 2
Book of Sayings Book 1
Book of Sayings Book 2
Book of Sayings Book 3
Book of Sayings Book 4
Scenar For Beginners

All books are available in print and eBook format from:
www.petazafir.com/books

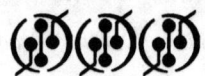

www.ingramcontent.com/pod-product-compliance
Lightning Source LLC
Chambersburg PA
CBHW071835290426
44109CB00017B/1830